# - CHC -
CERTIFIED HEALTH COACH

# LOVE
## YOURSELF
## TO LIFE

### NURSES'EDITION

## Lillie A. Hill
### RN, MSN, ACUE

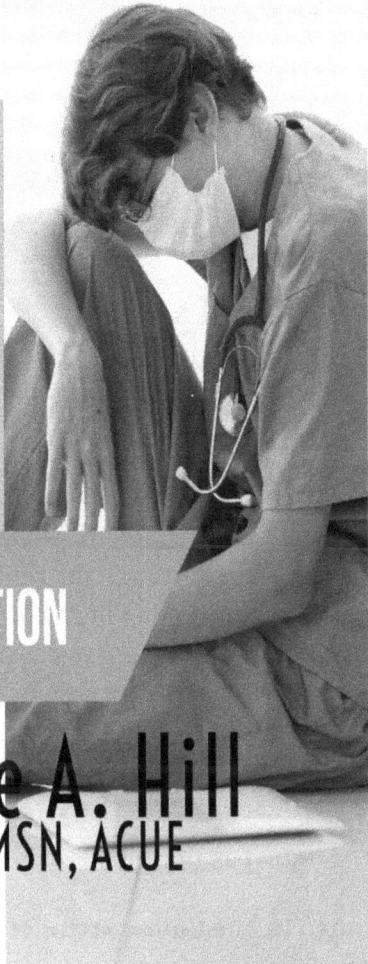

**Love Yourself to Life**
*Nurses' Edition*

Lillie A. Hill. Copyright © 2021

**EMPOWER ME BOOKS, INC.**
*A Subsidiary of Empower Me Enterprises, Inc.*

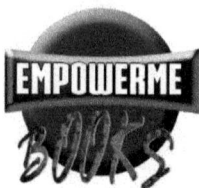

**ISBN: 978-1954418899**

**Printed in The United States of America**

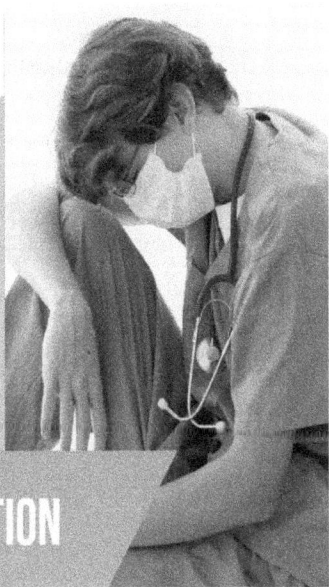

# LOVE
## YOURSELF
## TO LIFE

### NURSES' EDITION

# FOREWORD

BY Mark C. Hand

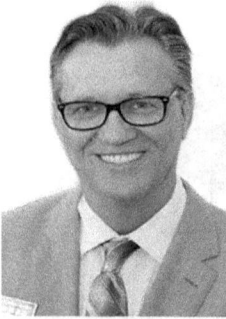

Linda. Tahisha. Mark.

These are nurses that dedicate their professional lives to helping others. This care often impacts their personal lives and wellness. Most of the time, nurses would say it is for the better - the field of nursing is exceptionally fulfilling. However, institutions are seeing increased reports of the opposite. Staff shortages, increased responsibilities, governmental regulations, and other job factors have contributed to nursing burnout and overall distress. Each of the nurse's stories depicted, by Lillie Hill, relates to the real struggles that nurses face today related to stress, burnout, and compassion fatigue. These terms are well-defined, and interventions are suggested to overcome anxiety, burnout, and compassion fatigue. Burnout, one of the six dimensions of distress, has many negative implications on both a personal and professional level.

Professionally, burnout can hinder job performance, change how nurses view their role and even put patients in danger. Personally, burnout affects demeanor, relationships, and overall quality of life. Nurse burnout is a widespread phenomenon characterized by a reduction in nurses' energy that manifests in emotional exhaustion, lack of motivation, and feelings of frustration and may lead to reductions in work efficacy explained by the author in Chapter 1. Each nurse's story depicts some of the signs and symptoms that nurses experience when faced with extreme stress. You will read what effects stress, burnout, and compassion fatigue have on nurses today and how they may promote better health and wellness.

Compassion fatigue is especially significant for nurses. Over time, it can profoundly impact a nurse's professional and personal life due to continual exposure to direct or secondary traumatic events. One intervention mentioned, by Lillie, in Chapter 2 is to "assess ourselves." It explains how to identify compassion fatigue and assess if any of the nurse's symptoms are described for the reader. Nursing is a challenging yet gratifying profession. Many of those who choose this extraordinary career do so because of a calling to help people. However, several factors have recently come into focus that has disrupted patient care and self-care balance. These include increasingly stressful work environments influenced by insufficient staffing, higher patient acuities, and patient expectations. Not only can these challenges erode a nurse's ability to provide quality care for patients, but for nurses to care for themselves. What happens to nurses when the day-to-day physical and emotional demands begin to take their toll? The information depicted in Lillie's chapters will help nurses make positive changes to their personal and professional lives. Well explained interventions are presented. As one of the quotes mentioned in Chapter 1, "I can be changed by what happens to me. I refuse to be reduced by it" by Maya Angelo, nurses can promote better health and wellness in their lives. These chapters in *Love Yourself to Life,* will guide the reader to better health and wellness.

**Mark C. Hand,**
Ph.D., RN, CNE
Clinical Associate Professor
East Carolina University

# FOREWORD

BY Gloria McNeil

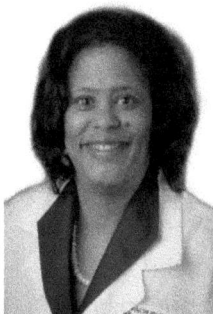

In the powerful words of Florence Nightingale, "With loyalty will I endeavor to aid the physician in his work and devote myself to the welfare of those committed to my care." I remember reciting this part of the Nightingale pledge and have worked tirelessly to live up to those words. I am honored to have enjoyed a successful nursing career. I have dedicated my life to caring for and taking care of my family, children, and the community. If given the opportunity to redo my career, I would still choose nursing. I believe I was born to be a nurse and have found that I enjoy giving to others and have unconsciously neglected myself at the expense of others. Nursing is a complex and noteworthy profession. We give more to others and find our strength and joy in helping others and often fail to care for ourselves.

The recent pandemic has given me an

entirely new perspective on life. I now recognize that I have minimal feelings of guilt for saying "no" and enjoying my "me time" doing whatever I need to do for myself. This book is an excellent reminder of the need to recognize the importance of self-care. The stories and examples described reflective behaviors that we nurses would not be proud of but do happen and can be attributed to burnout or stress.

I met Lillie in the early '90s. I watched her grow from a new nurse and then educator. She expanded her education and completed her Master's Degree in Education. Our paths crossed again when she was on faculty at a local university, and she invited me to speak to her student nurses. I am incredibly proud of Lillie for bringing this critical topic forward.

**Dr. Gloria A. McNeil,**
DNP, MA, MBA, RN, NE-BC, NEA-BC, CENP
Associate Chief Nursing Officer,
Duke Regional Hospital

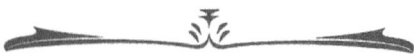

## DEDICATION

*This book is dedicated to all the amazing nurses around the world.*

*Nurses who can hold it all together with a roll of gauze and a pair of scissors.*

*Nurses who delegate and legislate.*

*Nurses who serve our country and the nurses who serve in our neighborhoods.*

*Nurses who make our hospitals and communities safer.*

*Nurses who cradle you for the first breath and who holds your hand until the last breath.*

*To these amazing men and women who dedicated their lives to making others' lives better,*
*I am grateful to call you colleague and friend.*

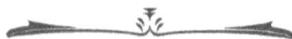

# ACKNOWLEDGMENTS

I first thank my *Father* above for allowing me to pen this literary work.

I am indebted to Empower Me Books for the professional support while creating and publishing this work. You helped me turn this dream into a reality.

I am grateful to Dr. Linda O'Boyle for instructing and mentoring me during my formative years in nursing school. She saw something in me that I did not, and if it had not been for her patience and grace, I would not have made it out of nursing school. Almost 25 years later, Dr. O'Boyle came back into my life and honored me with the blessing of being my colleague and friend.

I am grateful to Dr. Gloria McNeil for giving me my first job opportunity when I moved to Durham, N.C. Dr. McNeil paved the way for many young nurses, like me, to forge ahead in the nursing profession. She showed us that there are many roles in this profession and that we deserved a seat at the table. I was thrilled when she would visit my classroom of undergraduate nurses. Their eyes would be trained on her as she inspired them to be the best nurses possible!

I offer special thanks to my Pastors Earl and Dr. Wanda Boone of At His Feet Ministries International. The many prayers and phone calls were the foundation that kept me on track during this work. They repeatedly told the congregation that we are to be Ambassadors of God. I can only pray that I represent Him as well as they have. I love you, Pastors!!

I especially want to thank my parents Roger and Annie Williams. Neither of my parents graduated from high school. My Dad made it to the sixth grade, then needed to quit to help on the family farm. My mother made it to the tenth grade. Both of my parents encouraged their (Eleven) children to obtain an education, but always first and foremost to achieve wisdom from God. My Mom always wanted one of her daughters to be a teacher or a nurse. Through God's grace, her wish came true.

I am grateful to my children, Brianna, Justin, and William. They spent many days checking on me and reminding me to step away from the computer. You three are an inspiration and will do great things!

### *Most of all,*
I am indebted to my wonderful husband,
O'Dell Hill.  Thank you, my love, for always
believing in me, even when I did not.   Thank
you for always providing a soft spot for me
to land during times of disappointment.
Thank you for being the prayer warrior that
you are in our home.
**I look forward to continuing this adventure
with you !!!**

# CONTENTS

---

# CHAPTER 1

## *Intro to Burnout and Stress*

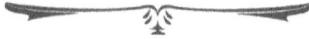

———— ✦ ————

*Linda C.*

*Ring. Ring. Ring!! Linda rolled her eyes to the ceiling as she checked her phone. If room 23 calls one more time, I am going to throw this phone out of the window! Exclaimed Linda. Just then, Linda received another call from the Health Unit Coordinator." Linda, the patient in room 12, wants to see her nurse. I asked if you could bring her anything, but she said that she just wanted to see you." I would like to see me too, Linda thinks to herself. OK, I love my job. I love my job, even with five patients on day shift, one no code, who is going downhill fast, one fresh post-op with too much blood on her leg dressing, two total cares (with a Nursing assistant who called out), and a patient with dementia who keeps wandering out of his room. As Linda is moving down the hallway, she is stopped by a Doctor who spits out post-op orders faster than she can write and disappears before she can repeat them. Finally, Linda, fully gowned in Personal protective equipment (PPE), steps inside of room 12, only to realize that the dressing supplies for the patient's wound are still in the clean hold. The phone rings again. Linda quickly steps to the doorway, removes her PPE, and answers the phone. "Hello, this is Dave from the lab. Ms. C in room 14 has critically low hgb (hemoglobin) and hct (hematocrit) levels. She is going to need to receive some blood. You need to report this to the MD STAT!" "Oh, just great," says Linda. I haven't eaten since last night, the cafeteria is closed, and I need to go to the bathroom. As she steps into the hallway, Linda glimpses a blur of silver hair, rushing to the elevator. NO! Stop MR. J, you can't leave the floor!*

*Linda thinks of her two young daughters at home, waiting to be carted off to ballet and gymnastics. I rarely get to see them, much less spend any real-time with them. John and I are more like roommates than husband and wife. I cannot remember the last time we went out to dinner or a movie. I wonder how much longer I can take this schedule. I cannot do another 12-hour shift. I became a nurse to make a difference and to take care of people. This is not what I expected. I just feel numb...*

*Tahisha L.*

*Ring! Ring! Tahisha rolls over and looks at the*

*clock. It is 5 am. "Hello," says Tahisha, she braces herself for the bad news." "This is Jody, the night charge nurse. I wanted to let you know that we have had two two nurses call out for the day shift, and there are no float pool replacements. We have a full house with 31 patients, and half of those are step-down patients." "OK, call the house supervisor and ask for extra nurses. "says Tahisha. "I will be there in 45minutes." Tahisha rolls over and covers her head with a pillow. Man, somebody should have warned me that Management was not all that it is cracked up to be. Upon getting to the unit, Tahisha braced herself for the disorganized chaos that seemed to invade her nursing unit. "Why can't I have one day when everyone shows up?" Jody meets Taisha at the door of her office. "We called a rapid response in room 18; the house supervisor says that there is no extra help and JACHO may be in the house today." Tahisha stepped into her office and closed the door. Leaning briefly against the back of the door, she exhaled deeply. I used to love this job, but now all I feel is numb...*

## Quote of the Day:
"I can be changed by what happens to me. I refuse to be reduced by it!"
Maya Angelou

As you care for your patients daily, you have probably thought about feeling stressed more times than you would like to admit. In nursing school, we are trained that stress can either be good (eustress) or not so good (distress). Eustress comes from positive events in our lives, such as getting a raise, earning a degree, or obtaining a job promotion. Of course, distress comes from those not so positive events: working too many shifts in a row, too many patients to care for, and organizational requirements that sometimes conflict with your ethics. Whether it is good stress or bad stress, our bodies are designed to react. According to Webster's dictionary, the most basic definition of stress is a state of mental or emotional strain or tensions resulting from adverse or very demanding circumstances. Some days I felt that my picture should be placed in the dictionary, next to this definition. As a Nurse, I learned early on in my nursing career that it is important to take time. I cannot be at my best and give my best If I am stressed out; however, there are periods in this nursing journey in which stress moves in and has its mail forwarded to your address.

What is most important is that you can recognize stress and how it displays itself in your life. Stress can display itself within four dimensions. Those dimensions include the body, the emotions, the mind, and the behavior. Let us explore how stress manifests itself in these dimensions. When we become stressed, our behavior changes, and we may begin to exhibit: a loss of appetite, an increase in smoking, become more accident-prone, and experience insomnia. Similar manifestations occur in our emotions. One begins to exhibit loss of confidence, apathy, irritability, and depression. Stress plays lots of tricks on the mind as well. Mental symptoms of stress include: excessive worrying, impaired judgment, nightmares, and pervasive negativity. Lastly, bodily symptoms of stress include headaches, muscular twitches, fatigue, and breathlessness.

It is often easy to explain these symptoms away as merely a response to a hectic workday or in response to a personal event. We are adept at putting our health on the back burner to continue doing the jobs that we love. As I mentioned earlier, our bodies are designed to react to stress, whether good or bad. We have an alarm system that causes us to either get into fight mode or flight mode. Both modes are considered protection mechanisms. Adrenaline pumps through our system, allowing us to react to the code blue in room 224 or to the active shooter, who burst through the ER's ambulance bay.

In either of these situations, our responses depend on how well our personal alarm system is working. As nurses, we encounter similar scenarios on a weekly, if not a daily, basis. Over time, we have adopted coping mechanisms to maintain a level of balance and peace. Nevertheless, what happens when the usual coping strategies no longer work, or worse, the coping strategy that we turn to, is not healthy, such as an increase in alcohol consumption, an increase in smoking, or inappropriate self-medication?

Unfortunately, unrelieved stress tends to escalate into a more profound syndrome, called burn out. This term has been used so frequently that it is sometimes used interchangeably with the words stressed out. However, burn out is a complication that occurs when our available coping mechanisms are no longer sufficient. According to Webster's dictionary, burnout includes physical or emotional exhaustion that appears to drain all motivation and strength from the individual experiencing it. Most often, it is described as a feeling of numbness towards life.

A nurse who is experiencing burn out is at a higher risk of making medication errors and possibly having an adverse patient event. We worked too hard to achieve our goal of becoming a nurse to allow stress and burn out to cause us not to be able to give the best care possible!

# CHAPTER 2

## Compassion Fatigue

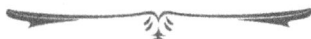

*Mark N.*

*This is my third hospice call today. I knew that Mr. X was close to death, but I am not ready for this today. Every time I go to that house, his stupid sons fight over their Dad's property. He isn't even dead yet! Don't they realize how precious these last moments are ??? His wife is trying to do everything that she can to help him live. If she wants to discuss one more thing that she found on the internet, I may lose it. She is very much in denial. I love helping and caring for the terminally ill, but lately, it has become more depressing. Every time I sit in the break room at the office, somebody tells me another heart-breaking story about their dying patient or the craziness that the family is displaying. I see death everywhere. Last week a twenty-eight-year-old woman died of breast cancer, leaving behind three beautiful children. I wish that I could adopt them. Gina and I have been trying to have a baby for five years, without any luck. The stress at work and home is becoming too much. The stress has become unbearable. Gina says that she is thinking about leaving me. She was my support system the entire time that I was in nursing school. I can't afford to lose her now. I definitely can't afford to take any more pain medications. I feel numb...*

## Quote of the Day:

*"We have not been directly exposed to the trauma scene, but we hear the story told with such intensity, or we hear similar stories so often, or we have the gift and curse of extreme empathy, and we suffer. We feel the feelings of our clients. We experience their fears. We dream their dreams. Eventually, we lose a certain spark of optimism, humor, and hope. We tire. We aren't sick, but we aren't ourselves."*
**Charles Figley**

Unfortunately, there is another area that is similar to burn out. It is called compassion fatigue. Caregivers who are exposed to traumatic stories and or situations repeatedly begin to empathize with the patient to the point of internalizing the actual symptoms. These caregivers often experience a type of Post Traumatic Stress Disorder (PTSD) by relieving these traumatic incidents each time they hear them. The term compassion fatigue is comprised of two very different words, compassion and fatigue. Nurses are well known for their compassion or sympathy. This is one of the foundations of nursing school curricula. The ability to "feel" the hurt of another individual and then be moved to action to resolve it is the epitome of what nurses display daily. We are trained to use our knowledge, skills, and abilities to alleviate the suffering of others. We are supposed to care for others, so then what is the problem? The problem presents itself in the word fatigue. Fatigue represents the opposing end of the health spectrum. As nurses tirelessly receive information, they then experience emotions that cause them to react. This cycle repeats itself repeatedly throughout a shift, day after day and month after month. Depending upon the work environment, our physical and emotional selves are called into action time and time again until we are drained and are no longer able to respond. Hence the term compassion fatigue means being unable to feel empathy for patients, families, and co-workers simply because that part of our spirit is weak and broken.

Sadly, it is while dealing with compassion fatigue that nurses began to contemplate leaving the profession. As the world is reeling from the effects of COVID 19, a deeper impact is being felt in the acute care centers, at the bedside. Day after day of caring for high acuity patients, patients who are gravely ill and possibly dying on their shifts, nurses are called, no expected, to render the most compassionate care possible, all the while worrying about their health and the health of their families. Healthcare workers are exposed to staffing shortages, policy changes, and other institutional restrictions that may play a role in advancing burnout and /compassion fatigue. Nurses experiencing compassion fatigue display a decrease in energy, a sense of helplessness, a feeling of disconnectedness, a lack of motivation, and personal and career dissatisfaction. These nurses also display deficiencies in their personal health and wellness, which can lead to a cascade of performance issues at work. Compassion fatigue is not a new phenomenon; even Mother Teresa understood the effects of it. She wrote in her plan to her superiors that it was MANDATORY for her nuns to take an entire year off from their duties every 4-5 years to allow them to heal from the effects of their caregiving work. (The American Institute of Stress)

As nurses, we are taught to use the nursing process to gather and analyze data regarding our patients' condition. The nursing process is a method of gathering data, interpreting it, and planning interventions to help our patients. Well, it is time for us to use this process to help ourselves. The first step in this process is that of assessment. We assess by asking questions or by looking for physical signs. We gain subjective data by asking questions, and objective data by looking for physical signs of a disorder.

Let's assess ourselves. How many of these do you notice during your workday?

- The ability to function is interfered with or altered.
- The situation or incident does not seem "typical or ordinary", it feels traumatic.
- "Compassion stress" impinges upon or breaks through normal boundaries
- Regularly waking up tired in the morning and struggling to get to work?
- Feeling as if you are working harder but accomplishing less?
- Becoming frustrated/irritated easily?
- Losing compassion for some people while becoming over-involved in others?
- Routinely feeling bored or disgusted?
- Experiencing illness, aches, and pains?

    Identifying one or more of these symptoms,

in your everyday work life can indicate that you are possibly experiencing compassion fatigue.

Although compassion fatigue and burnout are very real syndromes, experienced in the world of nursing, they do not have to bring an end to our much-loved careers. We are capable critical thinkers who can fix anything with a roll of tape and a pair of scissors! Nurses' this a wakeup call for us to unite and regain our health and wholeness.

As we look forward to positively impacting our lives and those of our patients, we need to ensure that we understand the terms health and wellness. These terms have often been used interchangeably; however, their foci are different. The term health typically refers to the abscence of disease or dis-ease. When individuals refer to being healthy, they begin to check off boxes regarding symptoms and or conditions. However, health is much broader than just the absence of disease. It is essentially an ever-changing process where an individual can achieve their potential in the (8) dimensions of health. Wellness is not viewed as the absence of disease or health issues but rather viewed as the highest level of health and wholeness. The dimensions of wellness are: Intellectual, Environmental, Social. Occupational, Emotional, Physical, Spiritual, Financial, and When we refer to wellness, we refer to the highest level of health possible in all these dimensions.

# CHAPTER 3

# *Intellectual and Emotional Wellness, Resilience*

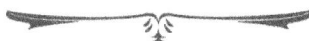

To do what nobody else will do,
a way that nobody else can do,
in spite of all we go through;
that is to be a NURSE.

-Rawsi Williams-

As nurses, we will have to return to that earlier resilience that existed as we persisted through nursing school. The American Psychological Association defines resilience as *"the process of adapting well in the face of adversity, trauma, tragedy, threats, or significant sources of stress."*

Stop! Let us focus on the part of that sentence: "the process of adapting well." What does that mean? We have been trained to adapt to the changes in our life and work environment. It is well known that if individuals do not adapt or do not adapt well, they will begin to suffer emotionally and possibly physically. Therefore, in order to enhance our personal resilience, adapting "well" must be our focus. Adapting well must be included in a structured plan. Better yet, a SELF Care Plan!

Just when you thought that you were done with those care plans, they boomerang back into your life !! However, the patient who is the focus of this care plan is you!! The most valuable person in the room. Remember that we are to put our masks on first!

So, Nurse up, and let's go!

As I mentioned earlier, there are (8) eight

dimensions of wellness. Humans are multi-dimensional beings, so it stands to reason that a multi-dimensional approach would be the most comprehensive. First, lets' get an understanding of each dimension.

### Emotional dimension:

A positive self-concept, which includes dealing with feelings constructively and developing positive qualities such as optimism, trust, self-confidence, and determination.

### Environmental dimension:

Good health by occupying pleasant, stimulating environments that support the well-being.

### Financial dimension:

Satisfaction with current and future financial situations.

### Intellectual dimension:

Recognizing creative abilities and finding ways to expand knowledge and skills.

## Occupational dimension:

Personal satisfaction and enrichment from one's work.

## Physical dimension:

Recognizing the need for physical activity, healthy foods, and sleep.

## Social dimension:

Developing a sense of connection, belonging, and a well-developed support system:
- A sense of belonging and a reliable support system to help during difficult times
- Make at least one social connection daily
- Do not hesitate to seek advice from peers and support groups

Now that we have an idea of what is in each dimension, let's begin to take a deep dive into each one. This is the part of the care plan where we are now planning interventions based on our gathered data about burn out and compassion fatigue.

## Intellectual Wellness

Intellectual wellness includes doing things that stimulate creativity and things that make us grow. How many of you have your daytime pattern so ingrained that you do not even notice? You get up at the same time every morning, check Facebook or Instagram, or some type of social media (back in my day, we read the newspaper). You eat breakfast, went to work, came home from work, fed the kids, took a shower, went to bed, only to get up and do it all over again the next day. I have pulled up into the driveway several times and said to myself; I do not remember how I got home... thankfully, someone was watching out for me. Our brain is an excellent tool, and it must be used and stimulated. Remember the old saying: if you do not use it, you will lose it."

Intellectual wellness also includes the ability to think critically and to allow our creativity to flow. Participating in mentally stimulating activities, such as reading a book, learning a new language, and doing a word search, can all be mentally stimulating activities. As a child, I loved to read. I would often get lost in a corner with the latest library book. My mind would be caught up in the latest plot or adventure. Sometimes, my Dad would take my library books and read them. He had a sixth-grade education but was one of the most intellectual men that I knew. I began bringing home multiple library books at a time so that we could enjoy our favorite pastime. Over the last few years, I have had very little time to enjoy reading. Of course, I read a textbook or a manual only to learn the material to teach others, but this is not as mentally exciting. Hmmm... I need a new hobby. Maintaining health within this dimension can lead to an overall sense of well-being.

### *Goal Activity Steps*

What are some ways that you can incorporate mentally stimulating activities into your day?

1.

2.

3.

Close your eyes. Think about things from your childhood that were fun for your brain. Was it creating poems, songs, or writing in a journal? Was it playing chess, cops and robbers, doctor, or perhaps you created your own games?

How about taking the intellectual challenge with me? Imagine a common ordinary ink pen. Now, I know that a nurses' pen is equal to all the gold in Fort Knox, and there is no such thing as an ordinary ink pen. You may end up sleeping with the fishes if you take a nurses' pen. However, play along for just a moment. How many different uses can you come up with for this item?

1.   A pointer
2.   A chart marker

Now it is your turn.

1.

2.

3

4.

5.

Great job!!  Way to be creative!

As nurses, we are utilizing our brains multitasking all day long. Quite often we do not get an opportunity to develop our intellectual wellness, in a way that is fun and effective.

So, let's mix it up a little bit and add some creativity to our lives!

## Emotional Wellness

**Quote of the Day:**
*"Calm mind brings inner strength and self-confidence, so that's very important for good health."*
*Dalai Lama*

Emotional Wellness or Mental Wellness involves the ability to recognize and cope with all our emotions, evaluate the feelings of those around us, and move forward with a positive outlook on life. As we focus on our emotional wellness, we begin to understand and respect our feelings, whatever they are. Often, we sell ourselves short by ignoring our feelings, especially if they are of sadness, guilt, or depression. Stuffing these feelings down inside of us and not addressing them can lead to deeper problems such as depression, anxiety, and even addictions. The truth of the matter is that our emotional wellness is more balanced when we pay attention to these emotions in the same way we do when we are happy or positive.

In order to address emotional wellness, one must learn and practice strategies of self-care. Repeat after me:

"Self-care is not a dirty word!"

We must put on our oxygen masks first before we can help anyone else. There are several strategies to be used for our emotional wellness, find what works for you, then repeat often.

1. Seek an experienced Counselor
2. Write three positive things that you notice, daily
3. Sit quietly, sipping a hot cup of tea
4. Put all electronics in time out for 10 - minutes
5. Practice Mindfulness or perhaps a prayer regiment.

6. Start a burnout support group on your nursing unit.
7. Work with a Health and Wellness Coach

Nedra Tawab is a licensed therapist and a relationship expert. She created the Self-care challenge: 30 Days of Loving Yourself. You can find her list at www.nedratawwab.com. After practicing some of these tips, you will feel brand new and unstoppable.

## **Goal Activity Steps**

1. Write a list of self-care activities that are appropriate for you.

# CHAPTER 4

## *Occupational and Environmental Wellness*

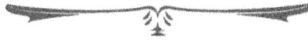

Maria finally had the opportunity to collect that urine sample from Ms. Jones   Dr. Flynn poked his head around the curtain. "Maria, can you check in the new patient that is in the lobby?" "Sure thing, thought Maria. Would you like me to clone myself as well? I am arms deep in catheterizing this patient, in the meantime, my bladder is about to explode". At that moment the phone in her pocket rings. Maria smiles as she ignores it. Maria hears her name being overhead paged. "Maria, there are urgent results being called in from the lab." The tech needs to speak with you." The clinic is especially busy today. Two nurses have been put on quarantine due to Covid 19 exposures. The patient was not symptomatic at the time. I guess that I am just lucky that I did not work with that patient. I really thought I would enjoy working in a clinic environment, but due to the number of patients *that must be seen and now adding all the new precautions due to COVID, it is overwhelming. To top it all off, I am not using my nursing degree in the way that I thought that I would. I love the patients and love my job, but things feel so overwhelming. I wanted to return to school to get my RN, but there never seems to be a good time. I need to keep this daytime schedule so that I can be available for my kids in the evening. Meals to prepare, homework to check, teacher emails to answer. As a single mom, there is no way that I can start going back to school with so much depending on me. Maria slips away into the breakroom. It is a windowless closet. She looks at the pot of plastic flowers on the table. The colors have begun to fade. She sits in a chair; after wiping off a clean spot on the table, she leans forward and takes a deep breath. "I love my job, I love my job, but today I feel numb...*

## <u>Occupational Wellness</u>

Howard W Thurman said, "Ask what makes you come alive and go do it."

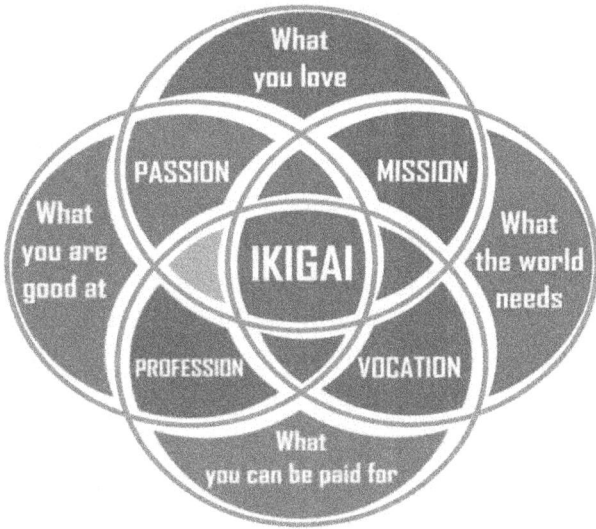

*Quote of the Day:*
*"Your work is going to fill a large part of your life, and the only way to be truly satisfied is to do what you believe is great work. The only way to do great work is to love what you do."*
*Steve Jobs*

Occupational Wellness involves being fulfilled within your chosen work or career path.

The term Ikagai has its origins in Okinawa Japan. Ikagai is loosely interpreted as a "reason for being." It is thought to be the thing that causes you to get out of bed in the morning. When you look at a diagram of this, you readily see four statements. What you are good at. What you love, What the world needs, and What you can be paid to provide. These statements are placed in four intersecting circles. The concept of Ikagai is achieved when these areas intersect in the four areas of passion, profession, mission, and vocation. Quite often, the profession of nursing allowed us to reach our "Ikigai". Nursing is a profession that checks a lot of the boxes. We can make a difference in others' suffering while belonging to a group of professionals and earning a decent salary. However, in times of stress and burnout, our reason for being stops feeling like a career and more like a coffin.

How often do you find yourself dreading Monday mornings simply because it is time to go to your job? Most people spend 40 hours or more a week at their place of employment. Some spend even more. Because we spend so much of our waking hours at work, shouldn't we at least enjoy it? Shouldn't we pursue revitalizing our Ikigai?

There may be many reasons why your current job is not your dream; however, you cannot let this kill your vision. What would your dream job look like, feel like? Is it fewer hours, a shorter commute, maybe it is time to be self-employed or return to school for another certification or degree? Does your current job allow for volunteer activities or child involvement leave (time to visit the kids at school or chaperone field trips)?

Maybe you are ready for more responsibility and want to move into a managerial role. Or, are you the one who loves to share your knowledge when staff and nursing students alike flock to your side? It is time to re-ignite your professional reason for being.

It is time to dream again. It is time to plan and implement interventions for your self-care plan. Create a vision board of what your dream career would look like. Add in all the details of income, position, etc. Also, address what it will take to get there—another degree or certification, special training, asking for a transfer, or starting your own business. In the middle of the vision board, set a target date for completion. A goal without a date is a wish. After you have created your vision board care plan, take the advice of Howard W. Thurman and, "Go do it!"

*Goal Activity Steps*
1. Create a Vision board of your dream career
2. Apply a specific date for achievement.

## **Environmental**

*Quote of the Day:*
*"One of the first conditions of happiness is that the link between man and nature shall not be broken."*
*Leo Tolstoy*

Environmental Wellness is when one maintains an awareness of one's environment and acts to preserve it. As I reminisce about my childhood days of growing up on a farm, I distinctly remember the smell of the grass, tobacco fields, and gardens with fresh vegetables growing in the sun. While in elementary school,

I had the opportunity to visit my brother, who lived in New Jersey. This was the first time that I had visited a big city. The sights and sounds were terrific. Skyscrapers reached the clouds, elevators, and people busily going about their lives 24hours a day. What a wonderful world we to live in, and to think we have the privilege of being able to leave this for future generations.

What could you do to improve the environment for the future? You can recycle, reduce your carbon footprint by walking, cycling, or carpooling. I am thinking about planting a tree to honor my loved ones. Whatever you do, keep in mind that you are investing in future generations.

As nurses, we need to immerse ourselves in nature and allow it to refill our souls. What does your work environment look like? Are you able to get outside and absorb some sunshine? How often do we teach our patients that sunshine helps to create Vitamin D in our bodies? Yes, we must be mindful of how much sun we allow on our skins due to other concerns. However, we certainly cannot teach something that we are not willing to do ourselves. Look at your workspace, are there plants or green spaces present? Are there pictures with nature scenes posted? A healthy work environment may include plants, but it also encompasses the office/unit's flow, the noise level and encourages a positive atmosphere for an employee's mood. How comfortable and clean is your breakroom? Maybe it is time to organize an environmental wellness committee !! Just make one change in your environment. The difference will amaze you.

## *Goal Activity Steps*

1. List 3 things that you can do to improve your work environment.

# CHAPTER 5

## Spiritual and Financial Wellness

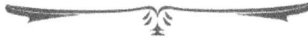

*Quote of the Day:*
*"Take the first step in faith. You don't have to see the whole staircase, just take the first step."*
*-Martin Luther King, Jr.*

Spiritual Wellness has been defined as the ability to obtain peace and harmony by living and connecting with our values. Lets' take a journey back to the days of being a nursing student. We were introduced to something titled "nursing diagnosis." These diagnoses were statements that we used as a professional to develop plans of care for our patients. One such diagnosis is that of Spiritual distress, as referenced by the North American Nursing Diagnosis Association (NANDA). The concept of

Spiritual distress is that an individual is experiencing an event that challenges their value and belief system. Patients may express anger at whomever they consider their higher power, concern about the meaning of life, or engage in blaming themselves for the illness. As we practiced holistic care and helped our patients deal with debilitating and sometimes terminal illnesses, we had an opportunity to witness the reconciliation of the illness through a spiritual lens. When these reconciliations occur, we see a shift from spiritual distress to spiritual wellness. Wellness in the spiritual dimension is equally important to us as nurses, as it is to our patients. When we clock in, we cannot check our spiritual selves at the door. As a matter of fact, our spiritual selves often help us deal, in a more compassionate manner, with the illness and hopelessness surrounding us. So, how can we address our own wellness in the Spiritual dimension?

As we think about our spiritual wellness, the focus is on developing the fruit of the spirit which will bring peace, harmony, and balance to our lives. One of the first activities is to take time to discover your values. If we do not know what we value, we are more likely to fall prey to everything that feels good to our senses.

Everything that feels good to us is not always good for us. Having values is what sets us apart from animals. Examples of values are courage, kindness, patience, integrity, gratitude, love, and forgiveness. Establishing balance in our values helps us to bring balance to our whole selves. After identifying your core values, prioritize them from 1 to 10, with one being the most important or non-negotiable. And ten being less important or possibly negotiable.

Keep in mind that event though your core values may remain the same throughout your lifetime; their level of priority may shift. Remember that as nurses, we must be in touch with our values and spiritual selves. I specifically practice being mindful in the form of spending time in prayer and in the presence of my Lord and Savior Jesus Christ. To clarify, this is what it means to me when I incorporate the 8 dimensions of spiritual wellness. This may be varying for you individually.

Here are some activates to try that will help restore your spiritual wellness.

- Take out time each day to reflect on your spirituality and core values

- Take the time to pray.
- Take a walk through nature and appreciate the beauty that is around you.
- Take the opportunity to give back or volunteer for a good cause
- Journal daily especially about the good things that happened to you.
- Seek a wellness coach and book a consultation with me as part of your list of wellness activities.

You can experiment until you find what works for you.

<u>*Goal Activity Steps*</u>
Write a list of interventions that you will use to enhance your spiritual wellness.

***Quote of the Day:***
***"An investment in knowledge pays the best interest."***
***Benjamin Franklin***

Financial Wellness is defined as the ability to be balanced in our financial lives, not just living to make money, but to be a good steward of our money. Whenever anyone questions me about what I do for a living, I sometimes cringe. Do not get me wrong, I truly love what I do; however, sometimes, the general public believes that by being a nurse, I must be financially well off. While serving as a faculty member in various Nursing programs, I have often heard this same sentiment from aspiring students. Yes, students have chosen this profession only due to the ability to obtain a specific financial status.

Nursing has afforded my family and me a satisfying lifestyle, but there have been times when lack of financial wisdom caused me to make some unwise decisions. Due to how I obtained my salary, my kids begin to act as if we had a money tree in the back yard. There were times when I would tell them that it took me a whole 2-3 hours' worth of work to obtain enough money for that internet game that they wanted. (*They just smiled and kept playing*)

I vividly remember the day on which I graduated from my master's degree program. I sat in the row of graduates and thought to myself; I now can finally reward myself with my dream car, a new Mercedes. I had planned on purchasing this car as soon as the ink dried on my degree. Oh boy, I could not wait to show up at work with this new car. While this daydream was wonderful, I had not sufficiently gained knowledge regarding the financial obligations that would come with it. At the time of graduation, I was a single mother, working in a salaried position for the state without the possibility of a raise. I had taken a significant pay cut to take this role to be available for my daughter, who was only in elementary school. In addition to this, the monies that I borrowed to pay for that degree would need to be re-paid.

Well, I learned a valuable lesson on the lot of the Mercedes Benz dealership. Always do your financial homework first! A few calculations readily told me that I was not ready for that type of car payment. I quickly develop a new dream, that of driving a car that has been completely paid off. With financial wisdom, planning, and the tenacity of my husband, we have achieved this multiple times. As nurses, yes, we can obtain a good salary, but then school loans become due. I have known nurses to have multiple jobs to live a certain lifestyle. They would leave a full-time role on Thursday to go work the part-time role on Friday through Sunday. No rest and more stress.

Today during a pandemic, there is the loss of

jobs or loss of income and an overall sense of worry regarding financial security. Nurses are consumed with credit card debt, school loan debt to the tune of thousands, and the never-ending stream of taxes.

Keep in mind that worries regarding finances can lead to the same amount of stress or burn out as being overworked or having a physical health condition. As an adult, I have always heard that a responsible person would plan in such a manner that they could leave an inheritance for his or her children's children. So. let's look at some ways to improve your financial wellness.

- Begin tracking your monthly expenses
- Start planning and live by a family budget
- See a financial advisor get a full view of your finances
- Review your benefits plan with a human resources representative
- Start an annuity plan with pre-tax monies (if you do not see it, you will not miss it)
- Start an emergency fund and do not touch it
- Start planning for retirement or repayment of college expenses

## *Goal Activity Steps*

1. What steps can you take to restore yourself to wellness in the financial arena?

# CHAPTER 6

## *Social and Physical*

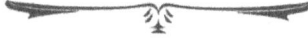

Social Wellness is about the ability to start and sustain positive relationships that add value to our lives and the lives of others. We are created to be social beings. During our times of stress, we reach out to friends or family to help ease some of our stress or distress. Having a good friend to rely on is critical in this day of fake Instagram friends.

Not only do we need strong friendships outside of the workplace, but we need them at the workplace as well. Granted, those workplace friendships grow from the camaraderie of facing work challenges together. I mean, let's face it when a patient is spewing explosive vomitus across the room, or you have just completed your fourth "Code Brown" in an hour, the only person who can understand this life is another nurse. More than likely, you will probably walk into the break room, where everyone is eating lunch, and start sharing in full glorious detail about the different colors of diarrhea and the various smells associated with it. We, as nurses, have a bond. Not only do we provide compassion and care for our patients, but we can come to the rescue of each other.

I remember working as the charge nurse on a medical-surgical unit. Most of the time, I would look at the schedule and cringe due to being short-staffed. However, I quickly learned that if "my gang" was assigned, we could handle just about anything. That is not to say that we did not have our challenges, but we knew that everyone on shift was there to work as friends, get the job done, and be a part of the team. Our team laughed and cried together. We celebrated marriages, new babies, wedding anniversaries, and college graduations. We knew each other's children, spouses, and sometimes parents. We were not designed to be islands or live in silos. We need that one or two friends who will take our secrets to the grave or will tell us the truth when we need it.

One day during a faculty committee meeting, the facilitator harshly rebuked me for whispering to another colleague. While feeling broken, fatigued, and very distracted, this public attack paralyzed me. I wanted to make her body disappear, but I had to repent of that thought. I abruptly left the meeting and ran to a coworkers' office. I cried uncontrollably for 30 minutes. This friend said to me. "It's time for you to do something about what you are going through. You are not the same person that you used to be, and it shows. You used to smile and love working with students, but burnout is written all over you. Even other co-workers have noticed the change in you." Darn, I thought that I was doing a great job, keeping my emotions hidden. Apparently, not! She then gave me the best advice ever. "It is OK not to be OK, but you should start seeing a counselor to get back on track."

I thought, who me, the person with years of experience teaching, the woman with a master's degree in Nursing, the Registered Nurse with 28years of experience, should see a counselor??? The answer to those questions was a resounding YESSS! Because I trusted her, and we were friends as well as co-workers, I was able to take her advice and began seeing a counselor. Because of her friendship, I was able to begin reversing the burnout and compassion fatigue that was overtaking my life.

Close your eyes, think about that one friend who is your ride or die. The one friend who knows what you are thinking during the staff meeting and causes you to burst out laughing. Social Wellness is about building and sustaining meaningful relationships. In our everyday lives, we each need that person who will go to their grave, carrying the secret of your real salary or the number of biceps curls you can do. So, close your eyes, picture that one friend who would fight by your side to the end. When was the last time you talked? What was one thing that you two did together that causes you to Roll-On-The-Floor-Laughing (ROFL) every time you think about it? Did you pull a prank on the residents or tape shut the manager's office door? OK, now after you get yourself together from laughing, wipe your eyes, go call that friend.

## Physical Wellness

Physical wellness is the ability to take care of our physical being. Exercise is good for the soul. OKAY, before you start throwing things at me, hear me out!

From the first day of grade school up until the present, we have heard how important it is to take care of our bodies. That adage, if you do not' use it, you will lose it has some truth in it. So, it should not come as a surprise that this dimension is included in our overall wellness journey. Also, physical activity has been shown to impact our emotional state as well positively. However, before you go out and pay for a gym membership (which I am not knocking. I had one before Covid 19 struck), let us look at non-conventional moving and active methods.

1. Have a dance party in your living room. (My husband and I grooved to Old Skool music for 45 minutes one day. It was a great workout!)
2. Walk your kids or pets around the neighborhood.
3. Do biceps curls with 2 Gallons of milk.
4. Drink green tea every day
5. Establish a walking group/partnership at work.
6. Incorporate wellness contests/walking meetings among your co-workers.
7. Organize different fitness challenges or groups (walking, hiking, running, biking groups, Fitbit, challenge.
8. Include 10-15 minutes of physical activity breaks throughout the workday. Push-ups, ergonomic stretching during breaks, Zumba on days off.

What creative way can you get active without equipment or spending money? Create a scheduled plan for getting active. Write this out on your calendar and go do it!!

Besides, physical wellness includes how we take care of our bodies. How often do we go through discharge instructions reminding our patients to exercise, eat healthier foods, drink 64oz of water, and have regular physical exams? As nurses, we know this routine so well that we can repeat it in our sleep. There is a big difference between knowing and doing. To increase our resilience emotionally, mentally, and spiritually, we must work at being our best in the physical realm. Here are some techniques to maintaining your physical wellness:

1. Schedule your annual physical
2. Schedule a prostate or mammogram screening
3. Investigate your wellness benefit available through your human resources
4. Incorporate self-care into your weekly routine
5. Obtain a Health and Wellness coach

How many times have you heard the saying that people in the healthcare field are the worst patients? We prioritize the care of everyone else before ourselves. We cannot give the best appropriate and prudent care if we are not caring for ourselves first. It is hard to pour from an empty cup. It is time to move, get active, get social, and crush it !!

# CHAPTER 7

## *Living Intentionally and in Full Expectation*

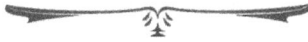

NURSE

EMOTIONAL

SPIRITUAL

SOCIAL

PHYSICAL

INTELLECTUAL

ENVIRONMENTAL

FINANCIAL

OCCUPATIONAL

## Poem of the Day:

## Greetings My dear Nurse
## by Brianna Forbes

*Hello, my dear nurse, welcome to work today*
*I love how you smile and wave good day*
*You are sweet, kind, and very hard working*
*I appreciate how you make it look easy*
*I notice you every step of the way,*
*you are the one whom I picked out of the crowd*
*You are my special nurse,*
*My special friend, indeed, you are!!*

*Dr. Q. Gerard, MSN, RN Nurse Faculty*

*"Dr. G, can't you give me an extra assignment so I may raise my grade to an A?" This came from the senior nursing student who was sitting on the other side of Dr. Gerard's desk. Dr. Gerard looks at the jar that sits on her desk. It has her favorite saying, "Ashes of dead Nursing students." She laughs to herself as she answers the student. "We do not give extra credit assignments in Nursing." "I am sure that with a little more study time, you will be able to earn a high enough grade to get that A." While reviewing the last exam with this student, Dr. G realizes that another student has similar answers and made the same grade. "Now,*

*I have to add tracking down cheaters to my to-do list', murmurs Dr. G. Just then, Dr. Brown, the Dean of the Nursing School, pokes his head around the corner and reprimands Dr. G for missing the faculty meeting this morning. Another student has submitted a grievance to be allowed back into the program. The same student who was caught cheating on every exam.*

*Doesn't Dr. Brown realize that this is the fourth meeting this week? And it is only Tuesday!!" Students cheating, committee meetings every day, precepting new faculty, and grading papers at home every night. I think that I am starting to get an ulcer. My 11-year-old son hates my job because I am always busy grading papers or on my computer. To tell you the truth, I am not so fond of it myself. My elderly mother depends on me, my son needs me, and my husband is doing the best that he can. I love teaching. Always have, but something has changed over the years. I feel as if I must fight everyone, the students, the administration, and my family, to have this career. "Is it worth it?" I don't know anymore" thinks, Dr. G. "I just feel numb…………*

## May 1986
*It was a beautiful day, sun shining, birds chirping, families smiling, and blue caps and gowns that*

*seemed to stretch for miles. It was graduation day!! It seemed as if this day would never come. I looked through the crowds and could see the smiles of anticipation on the faces of my classmates. We did it. We were finally graduating from nursing school, after many all-night study sessions, O' Dark thirty rides to the hospital for clinical and enough care plans to destroy a forest and to wallpaper the nursing building.*

*I was graduating with a degree in nursing. I vividly remember sitting in my favorite professor's office and listened as she told me that "Nursing is the hardest job that I would ever love." I smiled widely at her, all the while thinking, how could this be hard? It could not possibly be any more challenging than what I went through over the past four years trying to get this degree!! "Oh well, maybe she has to tell everyone that. My parents and all of my siblings were present for this day. I was on cloud nine and looked forward to a long, fulfilling career in nursing. I had been trained by the best with all the trade techniques to lead a long, happy life. I was thrilled and ready to begin a long love affair with nursing.*

<u>May 2018</u>
*I love my job, I love my job, I love caring for patients, I love teaching and I love being a nurse!!*

*I repeated this mantra as if trying to convince myself of this fact. It was taking a lot longer than usual to inspire those happy feelings of love and contentment. So far, this year has been a tough one, with one health crisis after another, my resilience was beginning to wear out. I looked out of the hospital window one day, while in clinical with students, and thought, wow is this all that I have to look forward to after 32 years of nursing?*

*Although I still loved being a nurse, something was different. The joy of serving was gone; I could not grade one more paper, give one more medication, nor sit in one more meeting. I smile as usual, but on the inside, I feel numb...*

*While continuing to stare out of the window, I hear my professor's voice. "Nursing is the hardest job that you will ever love." But this time, I heard a second voice," To continue enjoying this challenging job, you must pay attention to the signals, take care of yourself and avoid burning out." Burnout! How did I miss hearing these important words all those years ago? She was warning me about this phenomenon, but somehow, I missed it.*

*Okay, so, after loving, caring for patients, families, students, and colleagues alike, I found myself in this grey space, where there was no joy, color, and hope. This is a far cry from that optimistic young graduate, who nearly did cartwheels when she received her license in the mail to work as a registered nurse. What happened to that joy and love of nursing? The better question would be," How do I get it back ?????"*

Nursing is an incredible profession. Nurses perform in many roles such as Direct care providers, Managers, Executives, Educators, Researchers, and Mid-level providers. Traditionally nurses have been one of the most trusted faces in healthcare. In the 2019 and 2018 Gallop polls, Nurses were ranked 85% and 84%, respectively, with the highest honesty and ethical standards. Nurses receive years of education in classes such as Anatomy and Physiology, Biology, Nursing care of the child, Nursing care of the critically ill, Nursing care of the elderly, and Nursing care of the Community. All designed to fill us with the knowledge and skills for our professional roles. But as I look back on my nursing education, I somehow missed the class on how to care for myself or my colleagues. Yes, I know how to celebrate a birthday or how to encourage someone after a bad shift. However, what do you do when you look in the mirror and find no joy or life in your chosen profession; or the calling, that you love?

I never wanted to be a nurse in the first place. One day my sister, Brenda, told me: "You are smart enough to be a doctor, so you are going to college to be a doctor. Well, that was that! I just believed her and from that day forward my career goal was to be a doctor. I graduated from high school and went off to college to begin my medical school training in the fall of that year. After taking two years of courses, I was ready to begin my pre-med courses. While speaking with the college advisor, I quickly learned two things,

(1.) It would take another 6 to 8 years to complete med school and I did not want to be in college that long, and

(2). the college that I am currently attending does not have a pre-med program! How did I miss that little but extremely important detail??!!!

While reading my transcript, she suggested that I apply to the nursing program, my GPA was high enough, and all I would need was one summer school course. As a result, I was able to enter the nursing program that fall semester, and I have not thought about being a doctor since.

Over the years, I have relayed this same story to many nursing students. Nursing had to be and is my "Calling." However, in May 2018, I realized that my calling now felt more like my coffin.

Burnout and compassion fatigue are real. I realized that I couldn't stay here appearing alive, but dead on the inside. Nurses, we can't stay here. For the benefit of the ones we care for, as nurses, we must care for ourselves first! If you have ever ridden in an airplane, you listen to the pre-flight safety demonstration before the plane leaves the tarmac. Included in this demonstration are instructions on how to apply an oxygen mask in case the pressure in the cabin of the plane drops. The key point is that the parents who are traveling with small children must apply their own masks first. Being a mother as well as a nurse, I had a problem with this statement until I heard the remainder of the instructions. The purpose of putting on the mask first is so that you will be able to help those who cannot help themselves. BINGO!!!

In the Fall of 2018, through a good friend's advice, I began to seek help, I put my mask on first. Through counseling, I was able to begin seeing light at the end of the tunnel. As my joy returned, not just for nursing, but for everyday life, I began wanting to share this with other nurses. This is how "Love Yourself to Life" was born.

The compassion that I used to care for my

patients and students have now been focused on Nurses. I am on an awesome adventure to help those essential workers realize how important self-care is for their journey. While working under tremendously stressful situations, such as concerns over PPE, discovering a patient was COVID 19 positive after you had provided care for two days, and the oh so familiar routine of being short-staffed, nurses need assistance in regaining and/ or maintaining their resilience. Many healthcare organizations are incorporating such techniques as mindfulness training and mediation or quiet rooms into their strategic initiatives to address burnout and compassion fatigue issues. I even know of a Chaplain who has a tea party for the staff in a certain nursing unit. Lights out, calm music, fragrant tea blends all lead to a few moments of peace and restoration.

As a Certified Health and Wellness Coach, using the Eight dimensions of wellness, I have been able to have more conversations with nurses, female, and male entrepreneurs about self-care and its place in our lives. This is a journey and by no means have I arrived. I plan to expand my social circle so that more of us can walk through this together. Lets' begin loving ourselves back to life so that we can get back to loving our families, friends, patients, and profession.

Now another piece of our self-care plan is that of prioritizing. We gathered data on the 8 dimensions of wellness. Now, it's time to prioritize which area needs to be addressed first. If you remember from nursing school, prioritizing simply means to address the area that would cause the greatest suffering if not addressed first. Place a number 1 - 8 beside each dimension. Also, feel free to add your own dimension if need be. Place a #1 beside the top priority and #8 beside the area of least concern.

After identifying your priority dimension, it is time to set a specific, measurable, achievable, realistic, and timely (SMART) goal. Once your goal has been identified, then you must give it some GAS (Goal Activity Steps). Just like a vehicle will not move if it does not have gas, neither will your goal. In your self-care plan, you are to list the steps or actions that you will take to achieve your goal. It is important to answer the following questions:

1. What are your resources?
2. What things may hinder you from achieving your goal?
3. What is your date of achievement of your goal?
4. How will you know if you have achieved this goal?
5. What are your evaluation criteria?

9. How will you reward yourself when you achieve this goal?
10. What will you do if you don't achieve this goal?
11. Which dimension will you tackle next?

Always remember to keep moving forward and loving yourself to life! This is a journey, but we can live it intentionally and be full of expectation for a great future.

## The Love Yourself to Life 2019 Nurses' Conference

*Lillie looked at herself in the mirror for the last time. A gentle knock came on the hotel room door. "Lillie are you ready?' asked Brenda. "The participants have begun arriving. You can meet and greet them before we get started." This has been a journey to get to this moment thinks Lillie. Love Yourself to Life 2019, Nursing conference. Pastor always said that nothing that you go through in life will be wasted.*

***Quote of the Day:***
***And we know [with great confidence] that God [who is deeply concerned about us]***

*causes all things to work together [as a plan] for good for those who love God, to those who are called according to His plan and purpose.*
*Romans 8: 28 (AMP)*

The burnout and fatigue that I went through was awful, but if I can help somebody else with my message, then it will have been worth it. Lillie followed Brenda to the brightly lit conference room. The room had lots of colors and felt comfortable. Nurse Entrepreneurs filled tables, around the walls of the room, with their various products and books for sale. "It is good to see nurses branching out and finding joy in other areas", thought Lillie. Smiling, she went to meet some of the participants, while the Nurse DJ played upbeat background music. Brenda came and tapped her on the shoulder. "It's time to get started." After being introduced by the Mister of Ceremonies, Lillie took the microphone and smiled. "Welcome to Love Yourself to Life Nurses' Conference. The purpose of this conference is to give you techniques and strategies to strengthen your resilience against Burn out and Compassion fatigue.

As nurses, we are not strangers to these concepts, but we may be strangers to the self-care needed to combat these concepts. I am grateful that you chose to go on this journey with me.

I met a few awesome folks whose stories just resonated with me. Mark N. who is a hospice nurse and sees death and dying regularly, Linda C., who works on a busy Medical-Surgical unit often short-staffed and without the equipment needed to perform at her best, Tahisha L, who is the Nurse manager of a busy Orthopedic Surgical unit who has to respond to staffing issues constantly, Maria H, who loves her role in the clinic, but is getting weary, and Dr. G. a nursing instructor, who has a vase on her desk that reads "Ashes of Dead Nursing Students" I have been there done that!"

At some point in my nursing journey, I have walked in your shoes. I know what it feels like to love your profession but hate what it is doing to your life. So, I would like to publicly thank you for letting me help you learn how to Love yourself Back to Life!! Let's get to it!!" Lillie smiles and looks around the room. And so, the journey to wellness continues......

# BIBLIOGRAPHY

1. Substance Abuse and Mental Health Services Administration, April 2016. SAMHSA's Wellness Initiative: Wellness Community [Power Point Presentation] Retrieved from, www.samhsa.gov/wellness-initiative/eight-dimensions-wellness.

2. The American Institute of Stress, 2020. Compassion Fatigue. Retrieved from https://www.stress.org/military/for-practitionersleaders/compassion-fatigue.

# BOOK REVIEW

BY Linda D. O'Boyle

**"**

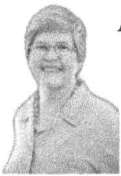

As a nurse educator, you often wonder if you make a difference for your students. Students do not often seem like they are paying attention during lectures and they are overwhelmed learning how to be a nurse. But after you have been teaching for over 40 years, you get to see your students "grow up" and become expert clinicians, leaders, and educators. Lillie Hill has developed into an outstanding educator who shares her experiences as a nurse in *Love Yourself to Life*. She has excellent recommendations to keep nurses professionally active with compassion. Nursing is a demanding profession. We must take care of ourselves in order to care for others. Lillie Hill recognizes the stresses we experience and has insightful recommendations to keep us alive and well as we practice our chosen profession.

Linda D. O'Boyle Ed.D., R.N.
Barton College

# ABOUT THE AUTHOR

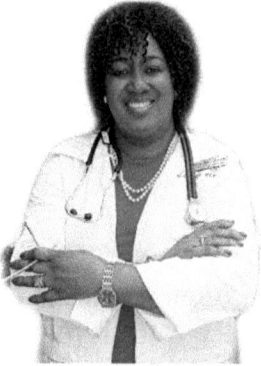

**Lillie A. Hill,**
MSN, BSN, RN, ACUE, CHC

While in nursing school and practicing as a nurse, Mrs. Hill believed that vulnerable populations were often left without an advocate.

On many occasions, she experienced that elderly and or minority patients were given health care information in a language that was not clear, consequently leading to noncompliance and more health complications. She believed that the best method to create a lasting change in the elderly and minority populations' health experience was to educate the next generation of nurses.

Mrs. Hill has been in the field of nursing education for over 23 years. During those years, she has had the opportunity to mentor and educate nursing students and Registered Nurses while instilling integrity, compassion, and caring.

Mrs. Hill obtained a bachelor's degree in nursing at Barton, in Wilson, NC., and a Master's Degree with a double major in Adult Health and

Geriatrics from Duke University School of Nursing in Durham, North Carolina.

Additionally, she is involved with various committees and has served as President-elect of the PI chapter of Sigma Theta Tau, National Nursing Honor Society.

She has also earned numerous awards, including The Excellence in Faculty Teaching award 2011 from Durham Technical Community College.

Mrs. Hill is the CEO and Owner of Health Education Solutions Inc, a company established to help improve the community's health through the vehicle of education. She specializes in Adult wellness, Caring for the Elderly, and educating healthcare professionals on how to avoid Burnout and Compassion Fatigue.

Mrs. Hill is dedicated to her students, patients, and the church community. Nursing has been an excellent vehicle that has allowed her to have a voice and to make an impact on the lives of those she serves.

www.Healtheducationsolutions.org
lh.healthedicationsolutions@gmail.com

## OTHER TITLES  BY THE AUTHOR

**Love Yourself to Life**
*Nurses' Edition Workbook*
*ISBN: 978-1-954418-99-8*

**Love Yourself to Life**
*Women's Devotional Journal*
*ISBN: 978-1-954418-98-1*

If you want to participate in the Love Yourself to Life
mentoring program, connect with Lillie on the web at
www.Healtheducationsolutions.org
and email her at
lh.healthedicationsolutions@gmail.com